I0479106

Long-lasting insecticide treated bed nets confer indirect protective effects against malaria in

sub-Saharan Africa

By

Samantha Smith

An Honors thesis submitted to the

Department of Biological Sciences

in partial fulfillment of the requirements for the degree of Bachelor of Science

Meredith College

Raleigh, North Carolina

May 1, 2020

Honors Student _____   Date: 05/01/2020

Thesis Director _____   Date: 05/01/2020

Honors Director _____   Date: 05/01/2020

Publication Agreement

I hereby grant to Meredith College the non-exclusive right to reproduce, and/or distribute this work in whole or in part worldwide, in any format or medium for non-commercial, academic purposes only.

Readers of this work have the right to use it for non-commercial, academic purposes as defined by the "fair use" doctrine of U.S. copyright law, so long as all attributions and copyright statements are retained.

Meredith College may keep more than one copy of this submission for purposes of security, backup and preservation.

Samantha Smith

May 1, 2020

Copyright 2020 by Samantha Smith

Abstract

The purpose of the project was to evaluate the indirect and direct protection conferred by community-level use of insecticide treated bed nets (ITNs) on occurrence of malaria in children under the age of five in sub-Saharan Africa. A total of 32 336 children under five were included in this cross sectional study of publically available Malaria Indicator Survey data collected between 2009 and 2017. Preliminary analyses identified confounding effects of household socioeconomic status, maternal education, urbanity, age of bednets, existence of standing water located near the respondents, and IRS use. For each country and corresponding year, the crude and adjusted odds ratios along with direct, indirect and total effects of ITN use were estimated. Neighborhood coverage levels of 50-100% and the use of an ITN prevented 8.1 (95% CI: 4.8 -11.1) cases per 100 children under 5, supporting the presence of protective total effects. The overall estimate of direct effects indicated that individuals who lived in a neighborhood coverage between 0-25% and 25-50% ITN coverage and were considered ITN users had a reduction of 2.9 malaria cases per 100 children compared to ITN non-users (95% CI: 0.9-4.7 and 0.7-4.8, respectively). Living in a neighborhood with 50-100% ITN coverage resulted in a reduction of 6.1 cases per 100 children for ITN non-users (95% CI: 2.7-9.7), supporting that there was significant indirect protection. Results for country and year specific data varied for total, direct, and indirect effects.

Key Findings

- The prevalence of malaria decreased across time for all countries and years.
- Direct protective effects were conferred for LLIN users living in a neighborhood where 0-25% and 25-50% of the community used an LLIN.

- Indirect protective effects were conferred for non-LLIN users living in a neighborhood with 50-100% LLIN coverage.

- There was a protective total effect for LLIN users living in the highest neighborhood coverage compared to non-LLIN users living in the lowest neighborhood coverage.

- Direct, indirect, and total effects varied between each country and years the survey was completed.

Background

Malaria is a mosquito-borne disease that causes flu-like symptoms that can lead to complications and become fatal. In 2016, the Center for Disease Control reported that 445,000 people died from Malaria out of 216 million cases worldwide.[1] This disease is especially problematic in sub-Saharan Africa for children, although control methods have increased in the past few decades. A common prevention method in use is Insecticide Treated Nets (ITNs), which can either be fabricated with the insecticide or treated every six months with insecticides. These act as a barrier while potential hosts sleep, and mosquitoes that land on the nets to feed receive a lethal dose of insecticide.[2] Another common prevention is the use of Indoor Residual Spraying (IRS), in which walls of houses are sprayed with insecticide. In this intervention, female mosquitoes receive a lethal dose when they land on walls containing the insecticide. Other methods include prophylactic drugs (PD), which are often given to young children and pregnant women.[2]

Several studies have evaluated the effectiveness of IRS relative to ITNs, with results suggesting that effectiveness of these interventions is context-dependent. One analysis of Demographic Health Survey (DHS) data indicated that IRS offered more protection against malaria infection among children under the age of five in Ghana.[3] In this study, ITNs only were protective in cases when the mother of the child had at least a secondary education.[3] An impact evaluation conducted in Rwanda on malaria intervention from 2000-2010 supported the combined use of ITNs, IRS spraying, and treatment of diagnosed malaria cases to reduce child mortality related to malaria from 58% in 2005 to 13% in 2010.[4] A meta-analysis of 30 studies comparing at least two malaria interventions including ITNs, untreated nets (UN), IRS, and PD, suggested that ITN use offered the most protection consistently (RR = 0.49, 95% CI: 0.32-0.74)[2]. In this analysis, PD, IRS, and UN did not show a risk reduction. Studies completed in various countries across Africa have supported the effectiveness of ITNs. In Malawi, a decline in malaria morbidity from 12.9% in 2011 to 5.6% in 2013 was attributed to a 20% increase in bednet usage among the population.[7] More specifically than ITNs, the use of long-lasting insecticide nets (LLINs) decreased the odds of contracting Malaria in the Democratic Republic of the Congo for children under five based off of 2013-2014 Demographic Health Survey data (OR = 0.72; 95% CI: 0.55, 0.77).[8]

In addition to the direct protection conferred, malaria interventions may also contribute to either protective or harmful spillover effects, meaning they will either further prevent malaria in the community or possibly increase risk of the disease for members of the community that do not use the intervention. In infectious disease settings, causal estimates related to intervention effectiveness can be biased in the presence of interference (also known as contamination), when the outcome status of one individual is associated with the treatment status of other individuals.[9] The presence of spillover effects (also referred to as indirect effects or herd protection) can lead to an over- or underestimation of the effectiveness of public health interventions.[5] With regard to malaria prevention, non-LLIN users could potentially confer herd protection in neighborhoods with high LLIN coverage. For instance, if LLINs successfully killed off mosquito vectors or reduced parasitemia rates among neighbors who used LLINs, then people within that neighborhood would have a lower risk of infection even if they did not use LLINs.[10] However, there is also a possibility that mosquitos may divert their feeding efforts from LLIN users to non-users. One diversion model suggests that malaria incidence increases for non-ITN users in areas where there is high ITN coverage, but low-killing levels. High LLIN coverage could then potentially increase harmful indirect effects for people that do not use an LLIN.[10]

Several studies have attempted to evaluate community effects of Malaria prevention. In Western Kenya, reduced rates of parasitemia and anemia were documented in a community that did not use preventative ITNs but was within 300 meters of a community with high coverage levels of (50-75%) ITN use. This finding is consistent with a positive spillover effect of outcomes associated with malaria. Lower levels of moderate anemia, hemoglobin level regression coefficient, and child mortality supported that ITNS provided some level of indirect protection. Although negative health outcomes associated with malaria were lowered, the actual prevalence of malaria was not.[6] Another example of protective spillover effects was supported by an evaluation of a randomized control trial done in Ghana's Kassena-Nankana district between 1993 and 1995.[11] This study evaluated the area 26 years after permethrin-impregnated nets had been used for an intervention trial. For every 100 meters between an intervention household and a control household, the childhood mortality ratio increased by 1.7% (95% CI: 0.6-2.6%).[11] Additionally, non-ITN intervention households that lived within 400 meters of ITN households did not have a significantly higher mortality ratio compared to ITN households (Standardized Mortality Ratio = 1.05, 95% CI: 0.79-1.40).[11] Although ITNs use is associated with both direct and indirect protective effects, concerns have also arisen about the decreased efficacy of bednets with age and the use of different types of insecticides. In a retrospective analysis of cross-sectional population data obtained from the DHS survey across 21 countries in sub-Saharan Africa, ITNs in general protected against malaria. Bed nets under the age of one year were deemed the most effective, and the magnitude of this effectiveness decreased as the age of the bednet increased.[12] Interestingly, the type of insecticide used on the net had no effect on the level of direct protection conferred.[12] A 2018 meta-analysis including studies done on ITN efficacy since 2000 indicated that LLINs were overall more effective in preventing malaria than ITNs, although both decreased the odds of malaria. LLIN users had 56% lower odds compared to those who did not use an LLIN, and ITN users had a 41% lower odds compared to those who did not use an ITN.[13] This study will investigate the direct and indirect protective effects of LLIN usage in the following countries in sub-Saharan Africa: Liberia, Malawi, Nigeria, and Uganda. Malaria outcomes based on a blood smear or rapid diagnostic test will be compared from 2009-2017 for both LLIN users and LLIN non-users.

Methods

Study Population

Data from Malaria Indicator Surveys (MIS) conducted between 2008-2017 from four sub-Saharan countries were included in this cross-sectional study.[14] The selection criteria used to identify these countries included the following: (1) countries geographically isolated to sub-Saharan Africa, (2) baseline malaria prevalence of at least 25 percent, (3) availability of GPS location data, and (4) availability of data from multiple surveys within the study period. Within these selected surveys, only data corresponding to children under five who were tested for malaria were included.

Variables

The outcome variable was defined as testing positive for malaria with a rapid diagnostic test (RDT) or blood smear. The potential confounding variables considered were chronic presence of standing water, wealth index, maternal education, urbanity, bed net age, and IRS use. LLIN use was defined according to survey participants' responses regarding whether or not the child in question slept under a LLIN the night before.

Neighborhood LLIN Coverage. Neighborhood LLIN coverage corresponded to the percentage of residents within a DHS cluster who reported using an LLIN the night prior to the survey interview. For each individual included in the survey, this percentage excluded him/her from the calculated measure. Neighborhood LLIN coverage was defined as an individual-level variable as
$$p_{ij} = \sum_{k=1, j\neq k}^{n-1} a_k/(n_i - 1)$$
, where a_k indicates whether or not individual k from neighborhood (i.e. DHS cluster) i reported using a LLIN the previous night, and $n_i - 1$ represents the number of residents within neighborhood i, excluding individual j. Neighborhood LLIN coverage was then categorized into three levels: low (0-24%), moderate (25-50%) and high (50-100%).

Statistical Analysis

Regression Models. In order to identify confounding variables, associations between potential confounders and malaria prevalence as well as LLIN use were evaluated for each survey using a chi-squared test. Generalized estimating equations were used to estimate coefficients associated with a random intercept logistic regression model, with fixed effects for individual LLIN use, neighborhood LLIN use and the interaction of both, along with covariates related to place of residence, household wealth index, age, maternal educational attainment, and presence of standing water by the household. DHS cluster-related random effects were included in the random intercept models for each unique DHS cluster across all surveys. All models made use of correlation structures that assumed independence among clusters. Pooled and stratified regression analyses were conducted using pooled and survey-specific data sets, respectively. Predicted malaria infection probabilities along with odds ratios and corresponding 95% CIs were calculated from parameter estimates obtained from the fitted models. All statistical analyses were conducted with R.3.5.0.[15] R code files used for analyses are included in the supplementary materials.

Estimation of direct, indirect, and total effects of LLIN use. Direct, indirect, and total effects of LLIN use were defined following Halloran and Struchiner (1995) and Hudgens and Halloran (2008), with predicted probabilities of infection estimated from fitted regression models (i.e. outcome model-based estimators).[16,17] Briefly, Let α represent the neighborhood LLIN coverage level, and a represent a binary variable that indicates whether or not an individual reported using an LLIN the previous night. $Y(a, \alpha)$ represents the average probability of testing positive for malaria for a given LLIN use category a and neighborhood LLIN coverage level α. Thus, $Y(a=1, \alpha = low)$ represents the average probability of testing positive for malaria for individuals that make use of LLINs and live in neighborhoods where the neighborhood coverage level is between 0 and 25%. Causal effects were derived from model predictions as follows. The estimated direct effects of LLIN usage within neighborhood coverage level α was defined as the risk difference:

$\widehat{DE}(\alpha) = \hat{Y}(0, \alpha) - \hat{Y}(1, \alpha)$, where $\hat{Y}(0, \alpha)$ and $\hat{Y}(1, \alpha)$ correspond with the average predicted probabilities of testing positive for malaria for kids that did not use LLINs and did

use LLINs, respectively, and lived in neighborhoods where LLIN coverage level α was either

low (<25%), moderate (25-50%), or high (>50%). Indirect effects were estimated as the risk

difference between LLIN non-users in neighborhoods with low vs. moderate and low vs.

high LLIN coverage levels, or $\widehat{IE}(\text{low}, \alpha) = \hat{Y}(0, \text{low}) - \hat{Y}(0, \alpha)$, where α represents

moderate (25-50%) or high (>50%) LLIN coverage levels. Total effects were estimated as

the risk difference between LLIN non-users in neighborhoods with low LLIN coverage levels

and LLIN users in neighborhoods with high LLIN coverage levels, or

$\widehat{TE}(\text{low}, \text{high}) = \hat{Y}(0, \text{low}) - \hat{Y}(0, \text{high})$. Ninety-five percent confidence intervals for these

risk differences were estimated via bootstrap resampling.[18]

Results

Prevalence of malaria and patterns of individual- and neighborhood-level LLIN use
A total of 32 336 children under 5 were included in data analysis methods which included

1303 DHS clusters. The overall prevalence of malaria from 2009 to 2017 in Liberia, Malawi,

Nigeria, and Uganda was 42.7% for children under the age of five. The prevalence of malaria

ranged from 25.4% to 52.2%, with Malawi 2017 at the lower range and Uganda 2009 at the

upper range (Fig. 1). The prevalence of malaria decreased in all countries across time. For all

countries and years combined, 45.1% of children under five slept under an LLIN the night

before the survey. The prevalence of LLIN users ranged from 29.9% to 76.1%, with Nigeria

2010 at the lower range and Uganda 2014 at the upper range. The percent of children that

slept under a LLIN increased over time with exception to Malawi. Neighborhood coverage

levels resembled patterns observed for individual LLIN use. The percentage of

neighborhoods with LLIN coverage between 50-100% increased over time for each country except Malawi, where the percent of the population who lived in a neighborhood that had 50-100% coverage decreased from 22.9% in 2012 to 8.7% in 2017 (Fig. 2).

Effects of individual LLIN use on malaria outcomes

For all countries and years combined, individuals who lived in a neighborhood coverage between 0-25% and 25-50% and were considered LLIN users had a reduced risk of malaria compared to LLIN non-users (Fig. 3). At the 0-25% neighborhood coverage level, there was a reduction of 2.9 cases per 100 children (95% CI: 0.1-5.6). At the 25-50% neighborhood coverage level, there was a reduction of 2.9 cases per 100 children (95% CI: 0.7-4.8). For the overall model, there was no direct protection for the 50-100% neighborhood coverage level for LLIN users (Fig. 3).

In Uganda 2009, LLIN users living in a neighborhood with 0-25% neighborhood had a reduction in malaria cases (5.5 cases, 95% CI: 0.1-11.2). In Liberia 2009, there was a reduction of 5.4 cases per 100 children (95% CI: 0.3, 10.9) for LLIN users in a neighborhood where 25-50% of the community used an LLIN the night before the survey. This neighborhood coverage level also was associated with direct protection for LLIN users in Nigeria 2010 (6.7 cases; 95% CI: 0.3-13.1). In Malawi 2014, there was a reduction of 8.8 cases per 100 children (95% CI: 1.5-15.7) at the 50-100% neighborhood coverage levels. For all other countries and years, there was no direct protection at any neighborhood coverage levels when comparing LLIN users to non-users. The probability of malaria in all neighborhood coverage levels was not different when comparing LLIN users and non-users (Fig. 4). However, the overall model supported that the odds of malaria was lower for LLIN users versus non-users for all neighborhood coverage levels combined (Fig. 5).

Indirect effects of neighborhood LLIN coverage on individual-level malaria outcomes

Overall for all countries and years combined, there was no reduction in malaria cases for LLIN non-users living in a neighborhood coverage between 25-50% compared to those living in a neighborhood with 0-25% LLIN coverage (Fig. 6). However, individuals that did not use an LLIN and lived in a neighborhood with coverage of 50-100% had a reduction in 6.1 cases per 100 people (95% CI: 1.0-11.7).

At the individual country and year level, there were no protective effects. There were, however, negative effects in Malawi 2014, Nigeria 2015, and Uganda 2014. LLIN non-users living in a neighborhood coverage between 25-50% had an increase in 6.7 cases per 100 children in Nigeria 2015 (95% CI: 1.6-12.3). Children living in Malawi 2014 and Uganda 2014 also had an increase in malaria cases at the 50-100% coverage level compared to 0-50% LLIN neighborhood coverage. In Malawi 2014, there were 13.0 more cases per 100 children (95% CI: 2.3-22.6), and in Uganda 2014 there were 10.2 more cases per 100 children (95% CI: 1.0-18.7).

Total protection conferred by individual- and neighborhood-level use of LLINs

There is a risk difference between non-LLIN users in low coverage neighborhoods and LLIN users in high coverage neighborhoods (Fig. 3). For all countries and years, there was a decrease in 8.1 malaria cases per 100 children under 5 (95% CI: 5.0-11.3) for LLIN users that lived in a 50-100% neighborhood coverage versus non-LLIN users that lived in a neighborhood LLIN coverage of 0-25%. At the country and year-specific level, there were no protective effects. However, in Uganda 2014 there was an increase in 10.6 cases (95% CI: 1.4-18.2) per 100 children under 5 for LLIN users living in a neighborhood coverage of 50-100% compared to non-users living in a neighborhood coverage of 0-50%.

Discussion

Prevalence of malaria and patterns of individual- and neighborhood-level LLIN use

The Demographic Health Survey, Malaria Indicator Survey data that is collected for each country is accompanied by a final report on malaria outcomes, LLIN use, as well as various other items that are included in the surveys.[14] Due to missing data that was needed to complete the adjusted analysis, such as IRS use, there are less children under five for this cross-sectional study compared to the original DHS data. For example, in Nigeria 2010, 1087 children were excluded from the original data set due to missing data. However, the malaria outcomes provided in the DHS report, as well as prevalence of LLIN use, were similar to this study.[14] Although the DHS final reports did not examine neighborhood coverage levels (Fig. 2), increased LLIN usage over time supports our report that the proportion of individuals living in a high LLIN coverage area of 50-100% increased over time. One exception includes Malawi 2017. The DHS reported that 67.5% of children under the age of 5 were LLIN users[14]; however, our data supported that only 31.6% of children under the age of 5 were considered LLIN users (Fig. 1). Upon further investigation, this discrepancy between data could be explained by the use of different variables to calculate the prevalence of LLIN users; the variable that the DHS used was for all ITN users, while the adjusted data set considered only those using a LLIN. Despite the difference between the reported LLIN use, the subjects that were included in our analysis had a lower prevalence of malaria as compared to all of the DHS subjects used for their final report.

Key trends for malaria outcomes over time were similar between DHS and adjusted data. The prevalence of malaria decreased across time for all countries in the adjusted data set (Fig. 1), and the prevalence of malaria decreased across time for all countries with exception to Liberia, whose prevalence of malaria stayed around the same from 2011 to

2016, despite an increase in the prevalence of LLIN users from 36.7% in 2011 to 43.5% in 2016.[14]

One limitation is that neighborhood coverage was defined according to DHS clusters, which consisted of a random selection of households within a randomly selected administrative unit.[19] Although clusters could be adequately considered independent of one another with respect to malaria transmission dynamics, assumptions related to within-cluster spillover effects could have introduced bias into our estimates. Approximate locations of DHS clusters are made available through the use of randomly displaced centroid coordinates; however, the exact locations of households within a cluster are unknown.[20] We assumed that individuals within a neighborhood were equally likely to be protected by their neighbors; however, this assumption fails to account for the effect of proximity to LLIN-using neighbors. Distance-based effects of LLIN use among neighbors may confound the relationship between neighborhood-level LLIN coverage and individual-level malaria status, as distances between households of one cluster likely differ across clusters.[21]

Effects of individual LLIN use on malaria outcomes

The adjusted model suggested that the odds of malaria was 13% lower for LLIN users compared to non-users (OR = 0.870, 95% CI: 0.760, 0.997) for all neighborhood coverage levels combined. A similar cross-sectional study evaluating malaria outcomes in 21 countries in sub-Saharan Africa between 2009 and 2016 supported that LLIN users had a 21% lower odds of malaria compared to non-users (OR = 0.79, 95% UI: 0.76-0.82).[12] This study also supported that the odds of malaria was not different for different brands of LLINs.[12] A meta-analysis of 30 studies, mostly consisting of randomized-control trials, which included data from 18 African countries, 11 Asian countries, and 1 South American country from 1988 to

2015, supported that the use of ITNs compared to no treatment reduced the rate of malaria

(RR = 0.57, 95% CI: 0.41-0.81).[2] However, this study included subjects from various age

groups and was not limited to long-lasting ITNs, whereas we aimed to evaluate malaria

outcomes only for children under five.

Interestingly, country and year specific data varied. Children under 5 in Uganda 2009

that were considered LLIN users had a 22.6% reduced odds of malaria compared to non-

users (OR: 0.774, 95% CI: 0.602, 0.996). However, there was not a reduced odds of malaria

in any other country or year (Fig. 5). A cross-sectional analysis of malaria outcomes in

Uganda was completed during a 28 month period following a mass LLIN distribution

campaign from 2011-2016. Out of the three regions assessed, only one had a reduced

incidence of malaria (aRR = 0.65, 95% CI 0.43-0.98).[22] Another cross-sectional study

analyzed malaria outcomes for children under 5 in Liberia using MIS 2011 data. Their

adjusted model, which included the child's age, gender, wealth, and urbanity, indicated that

LLIN users did not have lower odds of contracting malaria compared to children that did not

use a LLIN (OR = 1.05, 95% CI: 0.99-1.11).[23] Similarly, our adjusted model did not support

that LLIN users in Liberia in both 2011 and 2016 had a reduced odds of malaria compared to

non-users (Fig. 5). A study evaluating MIS data for Malawi 2012 and 2014 also supported

that the prevalence of malaria did not decrease across time in children under five despite an

increase in LLIN use, comparable to our model.[24] Their adjusted model suggested that

children who did not use an LLIN had an increased odds of malaria compared to non-users in

2012, but the odds were not different for LLIN users and non-users in 2014 (OR = 1.4, 95%

CI: 1.1-1.9 and OR = 1.5, 95% CI: 0.9-2.4, respectively).[24] They cited possible reasons for no

decrease in direct protection despite increased prevention methods, which included insecticide resistance, misuse of the LLINs for fishing on Lake Malawi, and the lack of knowledge on malaria prevention tactics from primary caregivers.[24] The misuse of LLINs for food acquisition may have also contributed to the decrease in prevalence of LLIN users from 2014 to 2017 (Fig. 1).[25] Contrary to our adjusted model, an analysis of the Nigeria 2010 data supported that individual child use of ITNs reduced the odds of malaria (OR = 0.79, 95% CI: 0.63, 0.99). However, the risk of malaria was only reduced in areas where a World Bank Booster Project campaign had taken place.[26]

Effects of neighborhood LLIN coverage on individual-level malaria outcomes

In an attempt to evaluate whether or not community bed net use affects direct protection conferred by LLIN's, malaria outcomes were analyzed for LLIN users versus non-users at 0-25%, 25-50%, and 50-100% neighborhood coverage levels. Based on the adjusted model for all countries and years combined, the use of LLINs was directly protective against malaria in neighborhoods where 0-25% or 25-50% of the population used a LLIN (Fig. 3). For both the 0-25% and 50-100% neighborhoods, 2.9 cases of malaria per 100 children under 5 were averted (95% CI: 0.1-5.6 and 0.7-4.8, respectively). At the individual and country year level, 5.5 cases of malaria were prevented in Uganda 2009 at the 0-25% neighborhood LLIN coverage (95% CI: 0.1-11.2). At the 25-50% neighborhood coverage level, 6.7 malaria cases per 100 children under 5 were prevented in Nigeria 2010 (95% CI: 0.3-13.1). Finally, 8.8 cases were prevented per 100 children under 5 in Malawi 2014 at the 50-100% LLIN coverage level (95% CI: 1.5-15.7). No other countries or years had protective or harmful direct effects at any level of LLIN neighborhood coverage. The overall model also suggested that the probability of malaria was not different for LLIN users versus non-users when analyzed at each neighborhood coverage level (Fig. 4).

For all countries and years combined, as previously noted, the use of LLINs was only directly protective when neighborhood coverage was 50% or lower (Fig. 3). This could potentially be explained by indirect protective effects. If non-LLIN users living in a neighborhood with high LLIN coverage exhibit herd protection, this could explain why there is not a difference in the odds of contracting malaria for LLIN users compared to non-users. On a smaller scale, the presence of community protection in neighborhood ITN coverage above 50% was seen in Western Kenya. Malaria outcomes, measured by anemia, parasitemia, and hemoglobin levels, were reduced for non-ITN compounds located near ITN compounds.[6] While this study did not directly measure LLIN indirect effects, results were similar with what we found comparing community LLIN use and malaria outcomes. For all countries and years combined, children that were non-LLIN users but lived in a neighborhood coverage of 50-100% had a reduction in 6.1 cases per 100 children compared to non-LLIN users that lived in a neighborhood with coverage between 0-25% (95% CI: 1.0-11.7) (Fig. 6). This suggests that there is some level of herd protection for non-LLIN users living in a neighborhood with high LLIN coverage, and could potentially explain why there was no direct protection at high neighborhood coverage.

Although the adjusted model with all countries and years suggests that non-LLIN users living in high neighborhood coverage levels confer indirect protection, indirect effects also varied among individual countries and years. The only indirect effects at this level were harmful (Fig. 6). In Nigeria 2015, there was an increase in 6.7 cases per 100 children under five for non-LLIN users living in a neighborhood coverage of 25-50% compared to 0-25% (95% CI: 1.6-12.3). Non-LLIN users that lived in a neighborhood coverage of 50-100% had an increase of 13.0 cases per 100 children in Malawi 2014 and 10.2 cases per 100 children in

Uganda 2014 (95% CI: 2.3-22.6 and 1.0-18.7, respectively) compared to non-LLIN users living in a neighborhood coverage of 0-50%. Increases in malaria cases among these specific countries and years could potentially be explained by mosquito diversion. One diversion model suggests that malaria incidence among non-ITN users is the highest in areas where ITNs cause high mosquito diversion when ITNs used by neighbors only kill 0-30% of the mosquito population.[10] This supports that the bed nets protected ITN users because the mosquitos were repelled from landing on the bed nets, but they were able to move to areas with non-ITN users and successfully feed and pass on the malaria vector to unprotected hosts. In contrast, in areas where ITNs killed 60-90% of the mosquito population, and therefore reduced their prevalence in the area, non-ITN users had a lower incidence of malaria compared to the low-kill areas. This suggests that some types of ITNS, which may include LLINs, may pressure mosquito populations to feed on more children that do not use LLINs due to this diversion principle if significant proportions of mosquitos are not actually killed by the LLIN.[10]

Total protection conferred by individual- and neighborhood-level use of LLINs

To our knowledge, no studies have been conducted evaluating malaria outcomes for LLIN users living in a high neighborhood coverage compared to non-LLIN users living in low neighborhood coverage. For all countries and years combined, LLIN users that lived in an area of 50-100% LLIN coverage had 8.1 less cases per 100 children compared to non-LLIN users living in a neighborhood coverage of 0-25% (95% CI: 5.0-11.3). At the country and year specific level, there were no protective total effects. However, Uganda 2014 did exhibit a harmful total effect. LLIN users living in a neighborhood coverage of 50-100% had

10.6 more cases per 100 children than non-LLIN users living in a neighborhood coverage of 0-50% (95% CI: 1.4-18.2).

Although the adjusted model suggests that all countries and years combined exhibit direct, indirect, and total protective effects, it is important to evaluate why these protective effects were not shown consistently across time and for each specific country. One potential reason for a decreased efficacy of LLINs is the increase of insecticide resistance in mosquitoes. *Anopheles gambiae* resistance has been documented for multiple types of insecticides in West Africa and pyrethroids in Liberia.[27,28] In Ethiopia, wild-caught mosquitoes had a reduced susceptibility to deltametrin, the insecticide used in some types of LLINs, after 26-32 months of use.[29] This further supports that LLIN efficacy decreases with age.[12,29] One suggestion to combat the increase in insecticide resistance is to once again consider the use of untreated nets.[10] Untreated nets are effective in reducing malaria morbidity, although most studies support that they are not as effective as LLINs.[10] However, their effectiveness should continue to be monitored as insecticide resistance continues to rise.

Another possible reason for inconsistencies in protective effects is that some mosquitoes' feeding times have shifted to earlier in the evening, when people are not protected by treated bed nets.[10] There is also variation in feeding habits, including the preferred feeding time, of *A. gambiae*, *A. arabiensis*, and *A. funestus* in sub-Saharan Africa.[10] This could potentially explain some of the differences between malaria outcomes in each country. The impact of climate change on mosquito ecology should also be further examined. One study's findings suggest that a gradual increase in climate temperatures could potentially allow *Anopheles* mosquitoes to inhabit areas of sub-Saharan Africa that were previously not suitable environments for their survival.[30] This could also lead to an increase in malaria prevalence in some regions across sub-Saharan Africa despite increased prevention efforts.

Along with differences in mosquito ecology, data may have been inconsistent between countries due to fluctuations in policies and mass distributions campaigns. For example, LLINs were only directly protective in Nigeria 2010 in areas where there had been a World Bank Booster Project.[26] Additionally, bed nets that are misused for food acquisition in Malawi could be due to a lack of enforcement on conservation efforts, and this could also lead to the decreased use in LLINs despite mass distribution campaigns. Despite declines in fish populations due to bed net use for fishing on Lake Malawi, people continue to misuse their bed nets in order to obtain food.[25] In the future, more studies should examine the association between country specific policies, distribution campaigns, and the efficacy of LLINs. It is still important to note that community use of LLINS conferred direct, indirect, and total protective effects on a large scale, and the prevalence of malaria decreased across time for each country included in the study. Distribution campaigns should continue, but efficacy should continue to be monitored across different neighborhood coverage levels and time.

References
1. *Parasites-Malaria*. 2018 [cited 2018 May 20].

2. Wangdi K, Furuya-Kanamori L, Clark J, et al. Comparative effectiveness of malaria prevention measures: a systematic review and network meta-analysis. *Parasites & Vectors* 2018; **11**.

3. Afoakwah C, Deng X, Onur I. Malaria infection among children under-five: the use of large-scale interventions in Ghana. *BMC Public Health* 2018; **18**: 536.

4. Eckert E, Florey LS, Tongren JE, et al. Impact Evaluation of Malaria Control Interventions on Morbidity and All-Cause Child Mortality in Rwanda, 2000-2010. *Am J Trop Med Hyg* 2017; **97**: 99-110.

5. Benjamin-Chung J, Abedin J, Berger D, et al. Spillover effects on health outcomes in low- and middle-income countries: a systematic review. *Int J Epidemiol* 2017; **46**: 1251-76.

6. Hawley WA, Phillips-Howard PA, ter Kuile FO, et al. Community-wide effects of permethrin-treated bed nets on child mortality and malaria morbidity in western Kenya. *Am J Trop Med Hyg* 2003; **68**: 121-7.

7. Escamilla V, Alker A, Dandalo L, et al. Effects of community-level bed net coverage on malaria morbidity in Lilongwe, Malawi. *Malaria Journal* 2017; **16**: 142.

8. Levitz L, Janko M, Mwandagalirwa K, et al. Effect of individual and community-level bed net usage on malaria prevalence among under-fives in the Democratic Republic of Congo. *Malaria Journal* 2018; **17**: 39.

9. Halloran EM, Struchiner CJ. Causal Inference in Infectious Disease. *Epidemiology* 1995; **6**: 10

10. Gu W, Novak RJ. Predicting the impact of insecticide-treated bed nets on malaria transmission: the devil is in the detail. *Malar J* 2009; **8**: 256.

11. Jarvis CI, Multerer L, Lewis D, et al. Spatial Effects of Permethrin-Impregnated Bed Nets on Child Mortality: 26 Years on, a Spatial Reanalysis of a Cluster Randomized Trial. *Am J Trop Med Hyg* 2019; **101**: 1434-41.

12. Janko M, Churcher T, Each M, Meshnick S. Strengthening long-lasting insecticidal nets effectiveness monitoring using retrospective analysis of cross-sectional, population-based surveys across sub-Saharan Africa. Scientific Reports: Springer Nature; 2018.

13. Yang GG, Kim D, Pham A, Paul CJ. A Meta-Regression Analysis of the Effectiveness of Mosquito Nets for Malaria Control: The Value of Long-Lasting Insecticide Nets. *Int J Environ Res Public Health* 2018; **15**.

14. *Malaria Indicator Survey (MIS) - The DHS Program.* 2009-2017 [cited 2018 May]; Available from: https://dhsprogram.com/What-We-Do/Survey-Types/MIS.cfm

15. Team RC. R: A language and environment for statistical computing. R 3.5.0 ed. Vienna, Austria: R Foundation for Statistical Computing; 2018.

16. Halloran ME, Struchiner CJ. Causal inference in infectious diseases. *Epidemiology* 1995; **6**: 142-51.

17. Hudgens MG, Halloran ME. Toward Causal Inference with Interference. *J Am Stat Assoc* 2008; **103**: 832-42.

18. Efron B. Bootstrap Methods: Another Look at the Jackknife. *The Annals of Statistics* 1979; **7**: 29.

19. ICF International. 2012. Demographic and Health Survey Sampling and Household Listing Manual. MEASURE DHS, Calverton, Maryland, U.S.A.: ICF International

20. Burgert, Clara R., Josh Colston, Thea Roy, and Blake Zachary. 2013. Geographic displacement procedure and georeferenced data release policy for the Demographic and Health Surveys. DHS Spatial Analysis Reports No. 7. Calverton, Maryland, USA: ICF International.

21. Jarvis CI, Multerer L, Lewis D, et al. Spatial Effects of Permethrin-Impregnated Bed Nets on Child Mortality: 26 Years on, a Spatial Reanalysis of a Cluster Randomized Trial. *Am J Trop Med Hyg* 2019; 101: 1434-41.

22. Katureebe A, Zinszer K, Arinaitwe E, et al. Measures of Malaria Burden after Long-Lasting Insecticidal Net Distribution and Indoor Residual Spraying at Three Sites in Uganda: A Prospective Observational Study. *PLoS Med* 2016; **13**: e1002167.

23. Stebbins RC, Emch M, Meshnick SR. The Effectiveness of Community Bed Net Use on Malaria Parasitemia among Children Less Than 5 Years Old in Liberia. *Am J Trop Med Hyg* 2018; **98**: 660-6.

24. Zgambo M, Mbakaya BC, Kalembo FW. Prevalence and factors associated with malaria parasitaemia in children under the age of five years in Malawi: A comparison study of the 2012 and 2014 Malaria Indicator Surveys (MISs). *PLoS One* 2017; **12**: e0175537.

25. Mwareya R. Misuse of Mosquito Nets Stressing Lake Malawi's Fish Populations 2016 *Yale Environment 360* 2016.

26. Kyu HH, Georgiades K, Shannon HS, Boyle MH. Evaluation of the association between long-lasting insecticidal nets mass distribution campaigns and child malaria in Nigeria. *Malar J* 2013; **12**: 14.

27. Namountougou M, Simard F, Baldet T, et al. Multiple insecticide resistance in Anopheles gambiae s.l. populations from Burkina Faso, West Africa. *PLoS One* 2012; **7**: e48412.

28. Temu EA, Maxwell C, Munyekenye G, et al. Pyrethroid resistance in Anopheles gambiae, in Bomi County, Liberia, compromises malaria vector control. *PLoS One* 2012; **7**: e44986.

29. Anshebo GY, Graves PM, Smith SC, et al. Estimation of insecticide persistence, biological activity and mosquito resistance to PermaNet® 2 long-lasting insecticidal nets over three to 32 months of use in Ethiopia. *Malar J* 2014; **13**: 80.

30. Afrane YA, Githeko AK, Yan G. The ecology of Anopheles mosquitoes under climate change: case studies from the effects of deforestation in East African highlands. *Ann N Y Acad Sci* 2012; **1249**: 204-10.

Figure Captions

Figure 1. The prevalence of LLIN use and malaria per country and year. Malaria prevalence decreased across time in each country. Malaria prevalence ranged from 25.4% to 52.2% in Liberia, Malawi, Nigeria, and Uganda from 2009-2017. The prevalence of LLIN users ranged from 29.9% to 76.1%, with prevalence generally increasing in each country across time, with the exception of Malawi.

Figure 2. The proportion of children under five living in neighborhoods with specified LLIN coverage. Overall, 35.8% of children under 5 lived in a neighborhood with 0-25% LLIN coverage. 35.1% lived in a neighborhood with coverage between 25-50%, and 29.1% lived in a neighborhood coverage of 50-100%.

Figure 3. Direct, indirect, and total protection conferred by LLINs in terms of malaria cases prevented per 100 children. For all countries and years combined, direct protection was conferred for children under 5 living in neighborhoods where there was 0-25% and 25-50% LLIN coverage. Indirect protection was conferred by non-LLIN users at neighborhood coverage levels above 50%. There was also a total protective effect.

Figure 4. The probability of malaria based on neighborhood LLIN coverage for both LLIN users and non-users. There was no difference in the probability of malaria for LLIN users versus non-users at all neighborhood coverage levels.

Figure 5. The odds of malaria for LLIN users compared to LLIN non-users. LLIN users had a 13% lower odds of malaria compared to non-LLIN users (95% CI: 0.760, 0.997).

Figure 6. The odds of malaria for non-LLIN users living in a neighborhood coverage between 25-50% and 50-100%. There were no reduced odds of malaria for non-LLIN users living in a neighborhood LLIN coverage level between 25-50% compared to 0-25% (OR = 1.00, 95% CI: 0.87-1.16). However, non-LLIN users living in a neighborhood coverage of 50-100% had a 25.7% lower odds of malaria as compared to non-users living in a neighborhood coverage of 0-25% (OR = 0.74, 95% CI: 0.63, 0.88).

Figure 1.

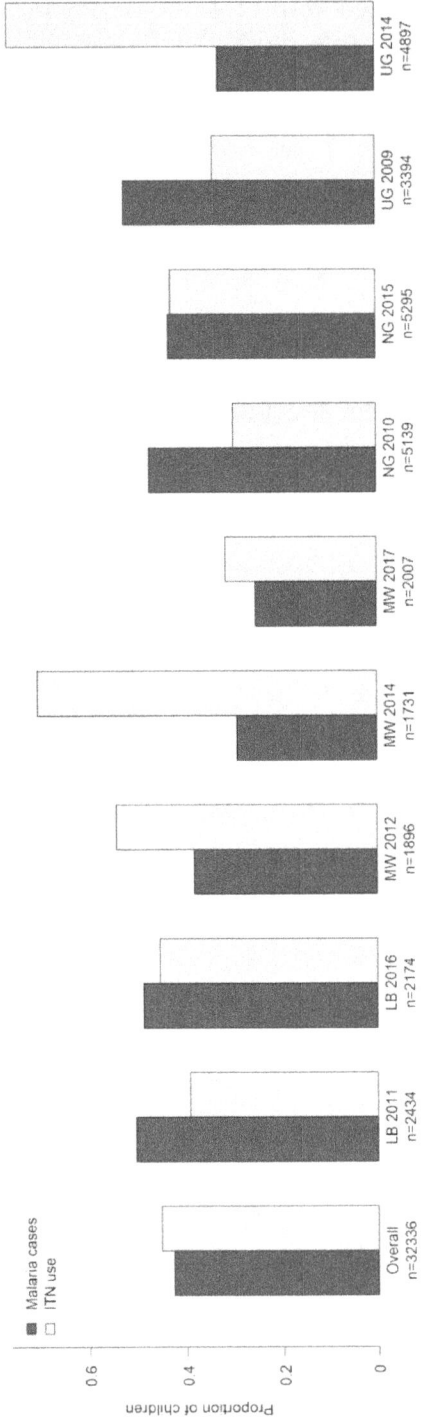

Figure 2.

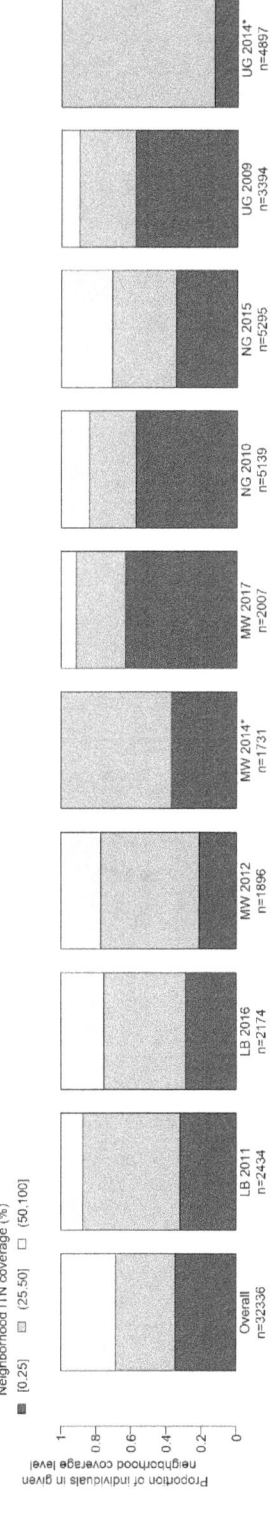

Figure 3.

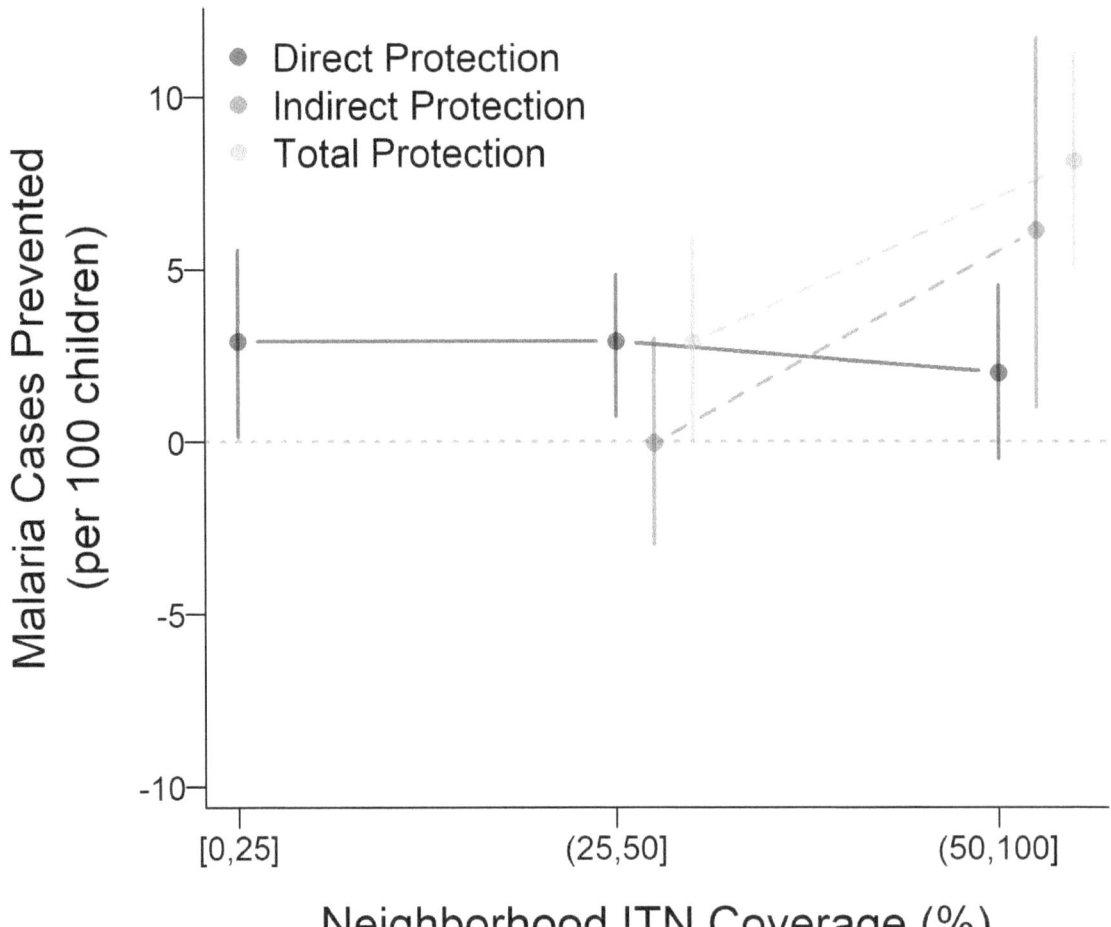

Figure 4.

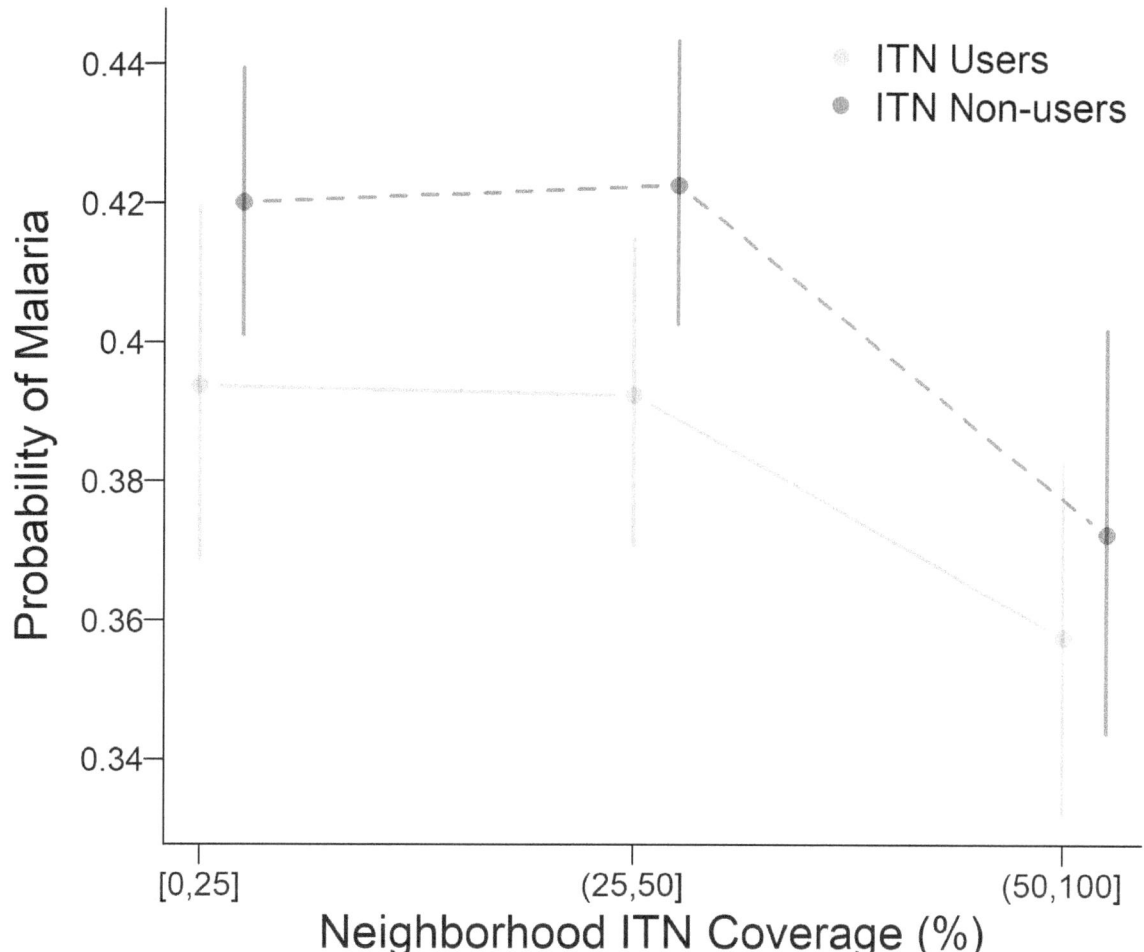

Figure 5.

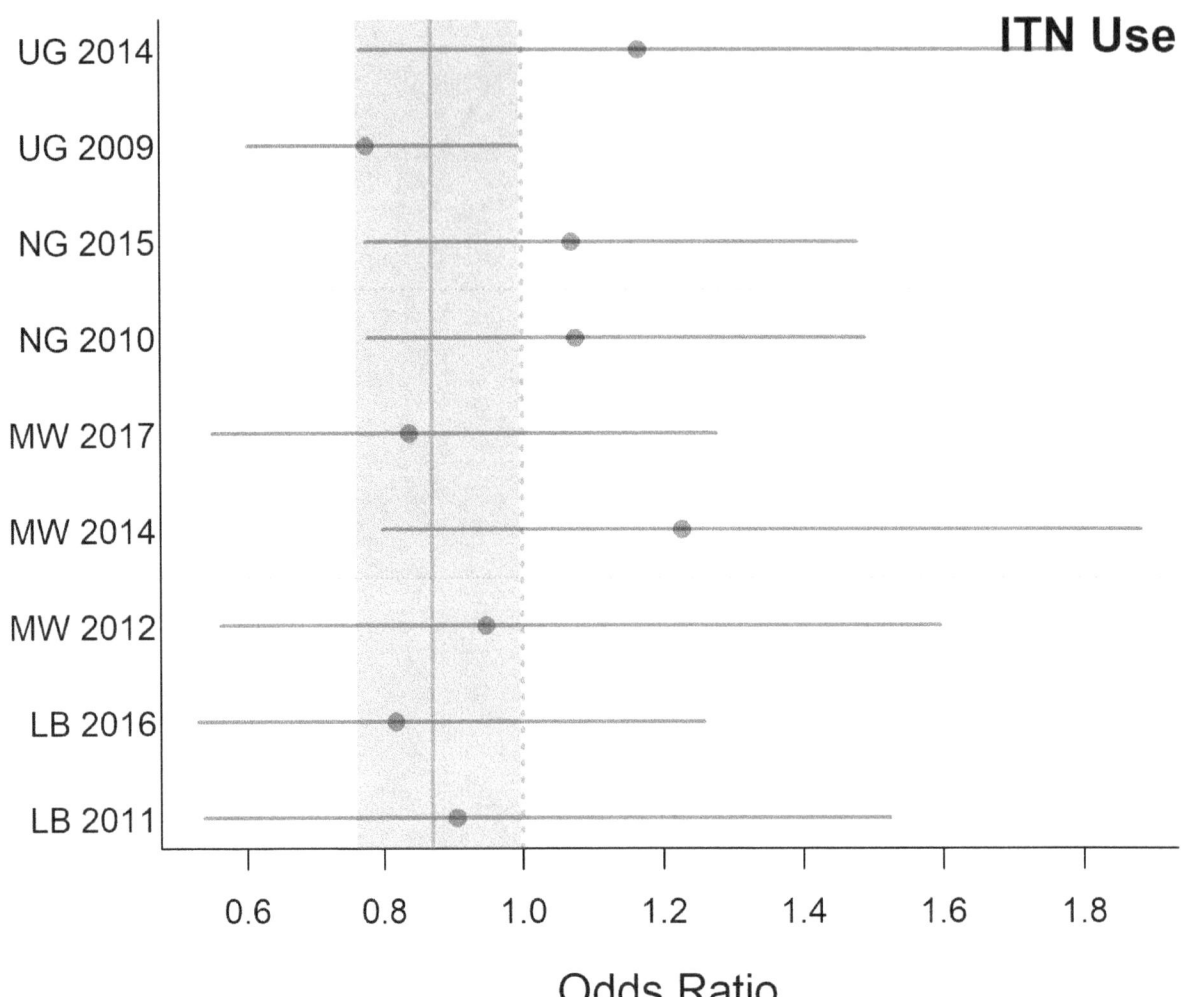

Figure 6.

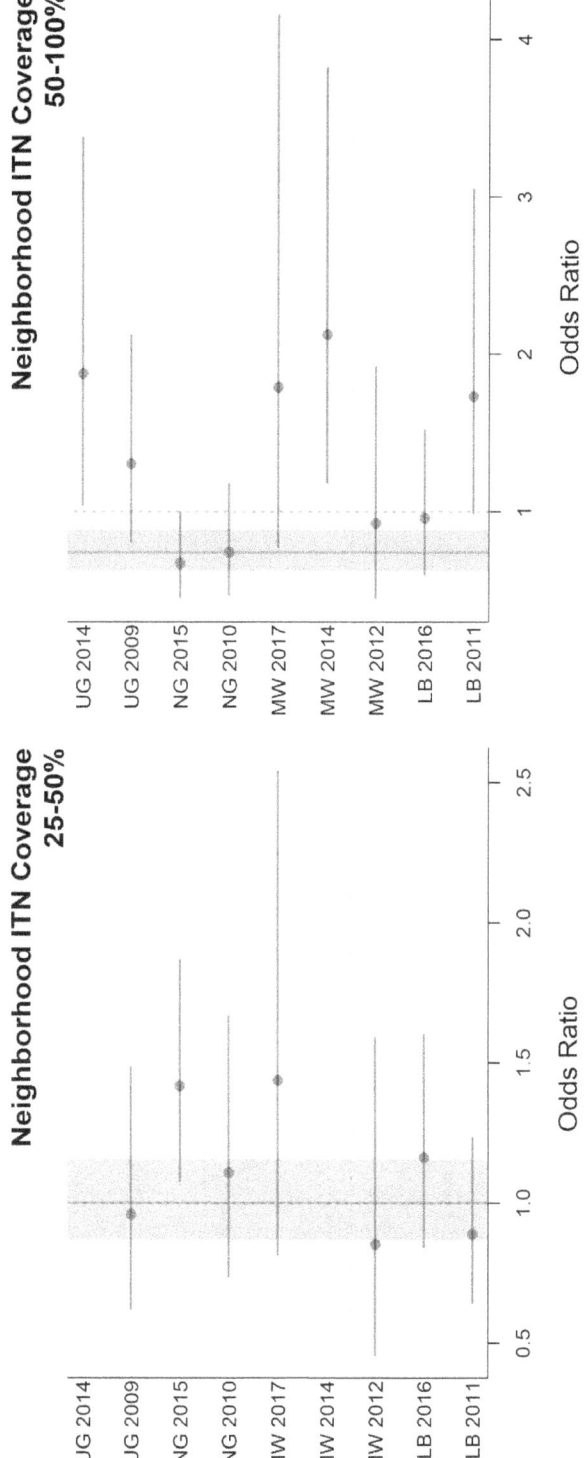

Appendix

Table 1. The direct effects associated with LLIN use based on neighborhood coverage levels.

Direct Effect (alpha)	0-25%	25-50%	50-100%
Overall	0.029 (0.001, 0.056)	0.029 (0.007, 0.048)	0.029 (0.007, 0.048)
Liberia 2011	0.021 (-0.087, 0.129)	0.004 (-0.047, 0.056)	0.048 (-0.049, 0.142)
Liberia 2016	0.040 (-0.041, 0.118)	0.038 (-0.020, 0.094)	-0.025 (-0.095, 0.045)
Malawi 2012	0.010 (-0.086, 0.111)	-0.037 (-0.098, 0.026)	0.028 (-0.056, 0.113)
Malawi 2014		-0.032 (-0.095, 0.040)	0.088 (0.015, 0.157)
Malawi 2017	0.023 (-0.029, 0.075)	-0.037 (-0.110, 0.030)	0.025 (-0.111, 0.179)
Nigeria 2010	-0.016 (-0.089, 0.054)	0.067 (0.003, 0.131)	-0.033 (-0.123, 0.053)
Nigeria 2015	-0.013 (-0.072, 0.047)	0.027 (-0.018, 0.069)	-0.042 (-0.089, 0.006)
Uganda 2009	0.055 (0.001, 0.112)	0.060 (-0.008, 0.127)	0.099 (-0.001, 0.201)
Uganda 2014		-0.023 (-0.090, 0.040)	-0.004 (-0.038, 0.034)

*The 0-25% and 25-50% neighborhood coverages were combined for Malawi 2014 and Uganda 2014 to improve estimates. The proportion of individuals living in a neighborhood coverage level of 0-25% was too low to estimate the direct effects.

Table 2. The indirect effects associated with non-LLIN users based on LLIN neighborhood coverage levels.

Estimate (0-25%, alpha)	25-50%	50-100%
Overall	0.000 (-0.030, 0.030)	0.061 (0.01, 0.117)
Liberia 2011	0.025 (-0.044, 0.096)	-0.115 (-0.237, 0.070)
Liberia 2016	-0.030 (-0.094, 0.035)	0.009 (-0.154, 0.109)
Malawi 2012	0.030 (-0.082, 0.148)	0.015 (-0.181, 0.251)
Malawi 2014	NA	-0.130 (-0.226, -0.023)
Malawi 2017	-0.052 (-0.144, 0.036)	-0.087 (-0.328, 0.030)
Nigeria 2010	-0.023 (-0.115, 0.070)	0.067 (-0.125, 0.192)
Nigeria 2015	-0.067 (-0.123, -0.016)	0.073 (-0.100, 0.111)
Uganda 2009	0.009 (-0.086, 0.105)	-0.056 (-0.197, 0.110)
Uganda 2014	NA	-0.102 (-0.187, -0.010)

*The 0-25% and 25-50% neighborhood coverages were combined for Malawi 2014 and Uganda 2014 to improve estimates. The proportion of individuals living in a neighborhood coverage level of 0-25% was too low to estimate the indirect effects.

Table 3. The total effects of ITN use for ITN users versus none users based on neighborhood coverage levels.

Estimate (0-25%, alpha)	25-50%	50-100%
Overall	0.029 (0.000, 0.060)	0.081 (0.050, 0.113)
Liberia 2011	0.029 (-0.044, 0.104)	-0.068 (-0.165, 0.037)
Liberia 2016	0.008 (-0.063, 0.077)	-0.016 (-0.107, 0.064)
Malawi 2012	-0.006 (-0.130, 0.111)	0.043 (-0.091, 0.168)
Malawi 2014	NA	-0.042 (-0.134, 0.051)
Malawi 2017	-0.090 (-0.160, 0.020)	-0.062 (-0.185, 0.041)
Nigeria 2010	0.044 (-0.057, 0.137)	0.034 (-0.073, 0.137)
Nigeria 2015	-0.040 (-0.102, 0.017)	0.031 (-0.036, 0.095)
Uganda 2009	0.069 (-0.030, 0.166)	0.043 (-0.079, 0.162)
Uganda 2014	NA	-0.106 (-0.182, -0.014)

*The 0-25% and 25-50% neighborhood coverages were combined for Malawi 2014 and Uganda 2014 to improve estimates. The proportion of individuals living in a neighborhood coverage level of 0-25% was too low to estimate the total effects.

www.ingramcontent.com/pod-product-compliance
Lightning Source LLC
Chambersburg PA
CBHW080423190526

45161CB00004B/266